# Wally

## Never Give Up

## Wally's Adventure With Asthma

By

Steven Noll

FIRST EDITION

ISBN:    978-1-952352-01-0


Published by:

# Crave Press

www.cravepress.com

## Dedication

This book is dedicated to my late father, Rev. Barry D. Noll (February 3, 1940 – January 13, 2012). I know you are looking over me and are proud of each of my accomplishments. Thank you for always being there for me and teaching me to be competitive and never give up.

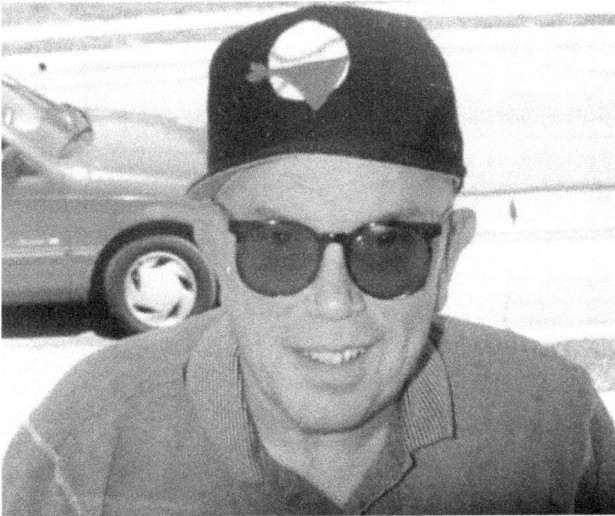

# Chapter 1

## The Adventure Begins

It was February 3, 1978, and it was Wally's father's birthday. His father was so excited. This year he was going to get a fancy cake from the local bakery. But Wally, who was yet to be born, had other plans for his mother while she was on her way to the bakery to pick up the cake.

On that cold, snowy day in February, Wally's mother went into labor. With all of her bags packed, Wally's mother walked to the front door. When she opened the door, to her surprise there were mounds of white in the blustery air. It was a blizzard, oh no! All of the cars parked on the tiny city street were snowed in. Wally's father shoveled the car out to make the trip to the hospital. Wally's two young sisters, nine-year-old Danielle and three-year-old Tracy, couldn't be home alone, so they had to take a taxi cab to their relatives' house three miles away. When Wally's parents arrived at the hospital, their car had a flat tire, so Wally's mother went inside while his father changed the tire.

Wally was born shortly after 1 o'clock in that afternoon. Instead of a cake for his birthday Wally's father was blessed with the birth of a baby boy. A bouncing baby boy he was not. Wally's delivery complicated. He was premature and wasn't supposed to be born for another five weeks. Wally had many health issues; his first breath was even a struggle. Luckily, the doctor was a military veteran that had dealt with difficult situations like this in the past.

The days ahead would be very tiresome and full of worry for Wally's family. Wally's mother was released from the hospital, but Wally had to stay in the neonatal intensive care unit (NICU), which is a special hospital unit for premature and ill newborn babies. The snow continued to fall, and Wally's mother had to take a taxi cab home when she was discharged from the hospital because the cars could not get out of the tiny city street where they lived. Because the street was snowed shut, Wally's mother was dropped off at the end of the street, and she had to walk to the house with all her packages from the hospital.

Several days after Wally was born, his family received a phone call from the hospital. Wally wasn't doing too well, and his family was supposed to come to the NICU. But the snow was still a problem. Wally's father had a boss that drove a large vehicle that could get through the snow, so his father called his boss to see if he could come to take them to the hospital. Thankfully Wally's father had an understanding boss, and he helped the family get to the hospital. Wally was struggling with numerous health issues, some caused by his premature birth. His lungs were not strong enough to breathe properly. Also, Wally couldn't breathe while drinking or eating, so he had to be fed with special IVs inserted in the top of his head. If that wasn't bad enough, Wally formed a blood infection called septicemia. While in the NICU Wally was diagnosed with the dreaded "A" word, asthma. With his health issues, he would have a long road to recovery.

## Chapter 2
## Growing Up

As Wally grew, his battle with asthma continued. Growing up as a young kid with asthma was difficult, not only physically, but emotionally as well. While other young kids played and joked, activities were different for Wally. Something as simple as a foolish tickle from his older sisters was a struggle. When Wally's sisters tickled him, his breath would get caught in his chest to the point he turned blue. His parents or sisters would blow in his face to get him to breathe again. It didn't take long for the foolish tickles from siblings to stop.

As Wally grew up and started elementary school, his adventures with asthma remained. He took many trips to the local hospitals after suffering asthma attacks. Wally was young and scared. His family was with him, but not being able to breathe was emotionally draining for both Wally's family and for him, too.

Wally was often absent from school because of his asthma. When he was in school, he was bullied because he was different than the rest of the kids. Other kids could be active in gym class, but Wally had limitations because of his asthma.

The technology and medication to treat asthma were not as advanced as they are today, and Wally tried many different medications in an attempt to control his breathing; however, the asthma attacks continued. Wally was on one medication for an extended period of time. It helped, but it had a side effect — Wally gained weight. With weight gain combined with his physical limitations led to more bullying.

Later in elementary school, Wally found a sport that he really liked — baseball. Wally's father found a local youth league that was willing to accept Wally even with his limitations. Wally's team was an amazing group of youngsters with great coaches. Even though Wally loved baseball, asthma got in the way. Wally found a position he was good at — catcher. But the combination of summer heat, long innings behind the plate, and wearing all of that gear meant some innings Wally had to be taken out because his asthma. Wally didn't let asthma take him away from the sport he loved so much. He did not give up; he kept pushing forward staying on the team and playing to his best abilities. Wally's team even won the championship!

In addition to baseball, Wally liked when his father would take him to see the fire trucks. Growing up in the city, there was often some kind of emergency that had fire trucks in the neighborhood. Each time, Wally's father gathered Wally and his sisters to go see the flashing lights and to watch the firefighters do their work. Wally took a liking to the action, but was often afraid of the firefighters with all their turnout gear. Wally thought of what it must be like to be a firefighter, but deep down knew his asthma would keep him from doing that job. Wally couldn't wait for the spring time when the fire truck would come to the school to hose the cinders off of the playground. During fire prevention week in October, all the school children would visit the neighborhood fire station which gave Wally an inside look of the fire station. They would see what life is like in the fire station from the fire trucks to the kitchen table everything looked so big. For now, all Wally could do is pray that one day his asthma would be gone so he could be one of those firefighters.

## Chapter 3
## Junior High Years

Wally couldn't wait to go to junior high. Going to junior high school meant being able to try out for football. Wally enjoyed playing football with his father. In August of Wally's first year of junior high, he signed up to try out for the football team. The process was very competitive and aggressive. In the summer heat in full pads, the team would do all kinds of workouts including a lot of running. It didn't take long for Wally to realize the hard truth — he couldn't play football because of his limitations due to asthma. What a bummer. Wally really wanted to play football. His father had played football for the same junior high, and Wally wanted to be just like his father. Wally's father didn't have asthma, though.

As Wally attended Junior High the bullying he experienced continued. Getting older, the bullying was worse; it was so bad, he switched schools. Wally went to school where his grandparents lived. The new school was awesome. They actually had real plates and utensils at lunch, not just plastic plates and utensils, and the food tasted like real food. Wally found some friends close to his grandparents' house, and he even got a newspaper route to earn some money. The kids at the new school were pleasant; Wally didn't have to afraid to go to school and be bullied anymore.

The following summer, Wally figured he would try out for football at the new school. The new school did things a little differently, and it wasn't so much running as his previous school so he could keep up with his teammates. The new coaches understood Wally had limitations. Wally worked hard and made the team, not as a starter, but he still made the team. His football playing ended halfway through the season, though. During pre-game warm-ups, one of his own teammates stepped on his hand, breaking his thumb. Wally had his arm in a cast for the remainder of the season.

## Chapter 4
## High School Years

Wally's high school years were met with more struggles with his asthma. His asthma was starting to impact things he enjoyed even more, he couldn't play sports in school anymore. He was absent numerous times because of his asthma, and more doctor visits meant more medicine to try and get Wally's asthma controlled. Wally went to see special pulmonary and asthma doctors who specialized in treating problems with the lungs like asthma. One doctor thought he had the plan that would help. In the back of the nasal passage is a tissue called the adenoids. The adenoids are supposed to help prevent illness, but Wally's adenoids were swollen and were not working properly which contributed to some of Wally's breathing problems. Wally went in for surgery to have his adenoids removed in a process called an adenoidectomy. With the removal of his adenoids this should help with breathing through his nose. Unfortunately for Wally, the procedure helped only a little bit.

Wally had some tough decisions to make as he progressed through high school. He continued to miss school a lot. Back in the early 1990s when Wally was in school, cyber school did not exist, and home schooling wasn't a popular alternative to traditional school. Wally's older sister Tracy found a correspondence school that offered a high school program to do at home. Wally made the decision to stop going to public school and to attend the correspondence school's high school program. Correspondence school was completed at home but without the computer technology. Correspondence school also didn't have the different grade levels like normal school; it was one big educational program. For each course, Wally would receive a shipment of books in the mail to study and complete assignments. Unfortunately, this meant no school sports, even if he could play, and no graduation ceremony for Wally. When he graduated, his high school diploma was mailed to him.

## Chapter 5

## The Ups and Downs and Not So Sweet Sixteen

Wally had dreams of getting his driver's license when he turned sixteen. Before he got his license, Wally's parents bought a gold 1970 Cadillac as the family car that Wally and his father were going to fix up. Wally still had his paper route, so he used his money to buy a chrome air cleaner for the motor to start fixing up the gold beast. Wally finally went to go get his driver's license. Wally was nervous having a state police officer sitting in the car next to him proctoring his driving test, but Wally passed his driving test on the first attempt.

Things were looking up for Wally. He went to a doctor that understood his situation. New medicine and technology meant that Wally could breathe better. The doctor told Wally that one day he would have his asthma under control. Wally would never grow out of asthma, but he could control it with medicine. This was amazing news for Wally and his family.

Then the emotional roller coaster started. As Wally was improving, his family members had health problems. Wally's grandmother was often in and out of the hospital with heart failure. One day when taking Wally's grandmother to the hospital for another heart failure episode, Wally's grandfather asked if he could also get checked out by the doctors. This was very odd because he had never been to the doctor except maybe once in his eighty years of life. The doctor did not have good news. Wally's grandfather had lung cancer that had progressed quickly, and his grandfather soon died.

Around the time of Wally's grandfather's cancer diagnosis Wally's mother suffered a traumatic fall. She slipped on the floor and hit her head around her ear on a shelf. This was a life changer for Wally's mother. She suffered damage to the inner ear that would stay with her for the rest of her life which meant constant dizzy spells. Luckily, Wally was starting to feel better with his asthma and he could now drive. He drove his mother to countless doctor appointments in the big city of Philadelphia, and he learned to drive on the Schuylkill Expressway at the age of sixteen. The Schuylkill Expressway is a multiple lane highway with congested traffic and angry drivers. Being a new driver, this kind of road can be challenging. If Wally could drive on the Schuylkill, he could drive anywhere. Wally didn't let the highway of a big city get him down; he drove with the confidence of an experienced driver.

The emotional roller coaster continued on a downhill track. Wally's father suffered a massive stroke which left him paralyzed on his right side and unable to speak. After spending time in the hospital and then the rehabilitation center, Wally's father was able to come home. Life was different for Wally. His father, whom he could always talk to, now couldn't answer him.

In October of that year, Wally passed the local volunteer fire station where they were having an open house for Fire Prevention Week. Wally thought about his desire to be a firefighter one day. In the back of his mind, he thought he could never fulfill that dream because of his asthma; however, he went back to his house and asked his parents if he could join the local fire department. Wally's mother was undecided for a bit, but she ultimately supported his decisions. Although Wally's father couldn't speak, Wally knew his father supported him. After some thought, Wally decided to become a volunteer firefighter.

## Chapter 6

## Learning to Live with Asthma

Wally was becoming a young adult and it was time to get a job. As Wally's asthma became more controlled with medicine, this meant more opportunities. Wally went to work in the local factory making batteries. Working in the local factory with summer heat didn't bother Wally's asthma. Being able to withstand these environmental conditions was a sign that his asthma was getting better.

Over the years, Wally was so accustomed to health issues of his own or taking care of other family members that he never put a lot of thought ahead in life; he lived each day by the moment. A new chapter would begin for Wally and at the age of twenty-two when he got married. Several years went by, and Wally and his wife were going to have a baby. This should be an exciting time for a young couple. Wally was excited, but he was also very concerned for the health of the new baby. He didn't want the baby to have asthma like he did. In 2005, their baby girl was born. She was healthy, and she didn't have issues like Wally. This was such a blessing.

As time went on, Wally's asthma became more controlled. He thought of the dreams from way back of being a firefighter. He was a volunteer firefighter, but he wanted to do this as a full-time job. He joined other volunteer fire departments just to gain more training opportunities and experience. It became apparent it was time to move forward in his career, and he left the factory for a job in a fire suppression company doing work on sprinkler systems and fire extinguishers. Wally was at the State Fire Academy and received a call from a local fire marshal with the news that he may not have a job when he returned because the company Wally worked for would likely close down. Sure enough, Wally arrived the following Monday morning to an empty office. He was without a job.

Wally didn't just sit around during this time of not having a job. He used this time to continue taking fire training classes and going for more national certifications. Five months went by, and it seemed he had found the perfect job. He was hired at the County Fire Academy as a fire service instructor teaching other firefighters. This was great for Wally. He got to meet so many wonderful people. Wally was truly passionate about the firefighter training and certification. Wally was as dedicated to firefighter training as an athlete is dedicated to their sport. He wanted to pass this passion and knowledge on, and he could do this by teaching others.

As Wally's health was progressing, his father's was not. One Friday night at dinner, Wally's father began to choke on ham. Wally had been training for years to save lives, but he never would have imagined having to save his father's life. Wally jumped into action performing CPR on his lifeless father. Wally was exhausted trying to save his father, and he didn't think he would be able to save his father. Miraculously, Wally continued performing CPR and his father started breathing again before the ambulance arrived. Wally never imagined all of his years of training would actually save the life of someone so close to him.

Time passed, and Wally's father began to experience greater health issues. His arm was swelled like never before. Wally told his mother to make an appointment with the doctor. Wally went with them to the doctor's office. From there, they went to the hospital for his father to get an ultrasound. Immediately after the ultrasound, they were told to go to the emergency room. The unthinkable was occurring, and they didn't know it. Wally's father had lung cancer. He died on Friday, January 13, 2012.

# Chapter 7

## Overcoming Obstacles

Wally spent his entire life overcoming obstacles. He overcame an obstacle that he and his family never could have imagined he would overcome. His asthma was no longer ruling his life; he was ruling his asthma. For years, Wally dreamed of being a career firefighter, a dream he never expected to come true. But training, hard work, and dedication paid off. Less than a month after Wally's father died, Wally was hired by a fire department as a career firefighter.

After being out of school for many years, Wally graduated from college while working full time and raising a family; he even became a member of an honor society. And now Wally finally got to attend a graduation ceremony.

While walking down the aisle to the graduation ceremony, Wally was overtaken by emotion; he finally did it. He has continued to push forward to advance his career.

Wally refused to let obstacles get in the way of his goal in life; after all, Wally overcame the biggest obstacle — his health. From that February snowstorm trip to the hospital to now, forty two years later, his life has been an adventure. His adventure is proof that you can overcome obstacles in life. No matter how far away your dreams seem to be, don't let go of them. Wally didn't, and neither should you.

## Acknowledgements

Ultimately, without the healing hands of God, all of this and my life would not be possible. This book would not be possible without the support of my family. I would like to thank my wife, Marci, and my daughter, Samantha. You have always supported me in everything. I would like to say thank you to my mother, Patricia; I don't know how you could be so strong dealing with having a child with such health issues. Thank you to my sisters, Danielle and Tracy, for dealing with me as a younger brother. I would also like to thank all of my friends that pushed me to progress along the way. I would like to finally thank Crave Press for believing in me and publishing this book.